Christoph Theissen

Long Covid Book

Christoph Theissen

Long Covid Book

Imprint
Christoph D. Theissen
Tilsiter Weg 15
41564 Kaarst
c.d.theissen@gmail.com

Copyright © 2024 Christoph D. Theissen
All rights reserved.

Except for use in a review, the reproduction or exploitation of this work, in whole or in part, in any form and by any electronic, mechanical or other means now known or hereafter invented, is prohibited without the prior written permission of the publisher and the copyright holder of this book.

Note: This book is based on my life story and the people mentioned are real people, so all names in this book, except my own, have been changed.

Foreword

I will never see the sea again. This sentence, which I once heard from an affected person, burned itself into my head and strengthened the hopelessness in me that I would never get well again.

I welcome you warmly and am happy you are here to accompany me through the most drastic part of my life story. I'll take you with me and tell you my story of my attempt to free myself from the quicksand, which only made me sink deeper with every desperate movement until I was finally unable to shower or take care of myself. I rushed from doctor to doctor in search of help until I ended up losing myself and yet in my darkest hours, I found my way to regain my health.

This book was written by me towards the end of my recovery journey and was originally never supposed to be published, as it is a personal reflection of the last two years and represents the conclusion of my illness for me. I am neither a doctor nor a scientist, my writings should not be seen as instructions or advice, but tell of my personal healing story, which I decided to publish because it can serve as inspiration for many sufferers.

Maybe you have affected yourself, then you should know that I know how you feel and what hell you are going through, which is almost invisible to others. But I believe you too can find your way to health, and I wish you all the best for your journey from the bottom of my heart.

Yours, Christoph D. Theissen

Table of contents

Chapter 1
The beginning   7

Chapter 2
Toxic self-help   12

Chapter 3
A trip to Hanover with earplugs and sunglasses   27

Chapter 4
Relapse but new hope   32

Chapter 5
An arduous path to the top   45

Chapter 6
New life   58

Thanks   64

Chapter 1
The beginning

In March of 2022, I was a busy man, in addition to my professional activity, I was always driven to look for a new business idea and only deal with things that would bring me money now or in the future. I usually felt my well-being and needs as an annoying evil that prevented me from fully pursuing my hunt for money and recognition.

My situation at that time was also not what you would call solid, as I had moved a few times within the previous months and no longer had a place to call home. The feeling of security that many people associate with their retreat had become alien to me. Since moving out of my parents' house, my apartments have changed as quickly as my working relationships.

From my perspective today, I would describe the said changes of residence as a hasty escape rather than being the search for a home.

After years of noise pollution that I had to endure in my condominium and that ultimately forced me to sell because I no longer had the strength to continue the fight, I just wanted to find somewhere to stay. Since the housing market already had a great shortage of housing in 2022, and my time for searching was more than limited, I was stranded in a small lightless basement apartment in April, not knowing that I would experience the worst hours of my life here.

However, I was in good spirits that my life would now slow down and calm down a bit, as I would now finally have peace in my home, which I so urgently needed to balance my job, which consisted of caring for an autistic child who used screaming as the only way to communicate. I was passionate about my work, but I felt increasingly burnt out by entering into conflict with a child on the verge of schooling for eight hours every day and getting into a rage again at home when the dumbbells of the gym shook the house below me again.

At this stage of my life, I felt an increasing irritability and what I would now call dysregulation in the body, but at that time I was not able to correctly interpret my body's warning signals. I had the habit of ignoring unpleasant feelings and always going beyond my physical limits, because for me, rest meant having to deal with my emotions and inner conflicts.

I am not clear about when I acquired this behaviour, but probably already in my early youth, so that over the years a large bundle of unprocessed situations accumulated, which cried out to be dealt with, but was masterfully ignored by me.

Although my body tried to tell me through different channels that something was wrong, I was one of those people who even managed to ignore the symptoms of tooth root inflammation until the tooth had to be extracted. The only thing I noticed more and more at that time was that I developed a susceptibility to infections.

Whereas in the past I was usually only really sick once a year, I now took every cold with me until I got sick almost monthly. I got sick, regenerated and got sick again a few weeks apart, my immune system seemed to be weakened. At the beginning of the year, I caught bronchitis that flared up again and again over weeks and did not seem to heal properly. I took sick leave and was prescribed antibiotics, which finally improved my condition.

On April 14, 2022, after this bacterial disease of the respiratory tract and my sick note, my first day of work at the special school began, which can be described as ordinary until the afternoon hours. After my break, however, I witnessed how one of the students injured himself on a disinfectant dispenser, whereupon an accident report had to be prepared. I was now sitting in an adjoining room and working together with Sascha, the special education teacher responsible for me, to document the incident. As we exchanged a few sentences, I noticed a feeling of restlessness spreading through my body and my mind wandering further and further.

"How exactly did the accident happen?" asked Sascha, who already noticed that my concentration was not focused on the situation.

At that moment I felt a real emptiness in my head, I didn't know exactly what had happened in my presence ten minutes ago. Nervous and insecure about my experience, I apologized to Sascha, who looked at me with a questioning look.

From this point on, my memory becomes blurred. I don't know what else happened at work, nor how I managed to get home, only that I arrived at my new apartment around 4 p.m. and went straight to bed from exhaustion. While I was lying on my bed and worrying about my cognitive deficits, I noticed that my T-shirt was already soaked with sweat, and my ears began to thunder more and more noticeably through my pulse. When I reached for the thermometer (my first thought was a relapse due to the infection), I noticed a temperature of 40.2 degrees Celsius, so I went back to bed and put the blanket over my head.

Unfortunately, the attempt to sleep failed miserably, as the fever was again joined by mental confusion, but this time it caused me less worry, as high fever is often accompanied by a fogging of the senses.

After a few hours of lying awake, I started to measure the pulse with my watch, as it was still racing, as if I was trying to climb a mountain on a bicycle, and indeed my count gave a heart rate of 145 beats per minute. I reacted frightened, of course, I had already gone through many infections in my life, and fever and palpitations were not foreign to me, but something about this infection felt different than anything I had known before. The strong physical symptoms, the strong fog in the head and especially the feeling of panic and fear. A few more hours passed, during which I remained almost motionless in bed, as every movement drove my pulse to unknown heights and I wanted to avoid unnecessary physical exertion.

I decided to go to the local hospital around midnight, but I was aware that I would not be able to make the journey on my own, so I decided to call an ambulance for the first time in my 31 years of life. In the phone call itself, I was met with incomprehension at first, until I mentioned that I suffer from shortness of breath. After the paramedics arrived, I went to the ambulance, where my high heartbeat and decreased oxygen saturation in the blood were detected, so I went to the hospital.

There I lay in the emergency room for some time and underwent various examinations, including a COVID-19 PCR test. In the morning hours, a doctor appeared and explained to me that I had a positive coronavirus infection and that my symptoms were caused by it. I should take it easy and consult a doctor if shortness of breath recurs.

Back home, I asked a relative around 8 a.m. to let me know about my work and went to bed exhausted. Nine days now passed, in which I alternated between phases of fever, chills and a strong fog in the brain, but what bothered me most was that I could not sleep, my day and night rhythm seemed to be completely out of control. I felt endlessly exhausted and yet so excited that every little movement or sound triggered a kind of adrenaline rush in me.

A small crack of the bed or the singing of a bird was enough to startle me, although I felt endless tiredness inside. I tried to kill my time with videos and activities such as puzzles, but after a few minutes, I had to realize that I lost all interest in the film I was watching and that doing puzzles overwhelmed my cognitive abilities, without being able to suspect that this state would soon be an integral part of my life. On the eleventh day after my positive test result, all flu-like symptoms receded. I felt drained, but happy that the stripes on my rapid test were only faintly pronounced, and was in good spirits that my sleep would also find a normal rhythm again, now that the fever had subsided.

I planned to go back to work the following Monday, and since, as mentioned at the beginning of my story, I liked to ignore the needs of my body, I also planned to start my dumbbell training again the next day. This behaviour can probably be described as irresponsible, but at that time in my life, the training was more of a compulsion than a health-promoting measure. The thought of not being able to train and thus losing muscle always put me in a bad mood.

So it happened that the next day, although I was still slightly positive, I built up my dumbbells and began to warm up my muscles. I noticed that my hands felt cold, as did my feet like an ice cube. I began to think about whether it was a coincidence or whether I was suffering from some kind of circulatory disorder, after all, I once read an article that described how COVID could change the structure and flexibility of blood cells. My body was the human equivalent of a radiator, I never suffered from cold limbs. I took off my socks and found that my feet had turned blue.

I was startled by the sight that presented itself to me and staggered a little. My entire circulation felt weak and vulnerable. I had the feeling that my brain was not supplied with enough blood. Everything was numb and strange. I decided, despite all the abnormalities, to continue my training.

Sport is good for blood circulation and if I train now, everything will settle down again, I told myself positively, although I was already enormously stressed inside and feelings of anxiety arose in me.

Chapter 2
Toxic self-help

Dogged as usual, I lifted the weights towards the ceiling with all my strength during the bench press, which I managed well, but when I finally finished my set, my pulse shot up like my barbell before. As an athlete, I was used to the heart working, but something was different than before. Every single blow was like thunder, permeated my body and was felt on my shoulder blades. I decided to stop my training and leave my apartment after a short break.

Still amazed and unsettled by the pulse noise in my ear, I went outside the door for the first time in twelve days. When I left the apartment, I noticed a change in my perception: the sun seemed to be unnaturally glaring, and my eyes seemed unable to fix on objects further away.

After a few steps, I felt an insecurity rising in me. I felt like a foreign body in an outside world that was hostile to me and decided to turn around on the spot. With a hint of a slight panic, I opened my apartment door and took a look in the mirror that adorned my hallway. In the reflection, I saw a pale man with reddened eyes and beads of sweat on his forehead. Although the fever had subsided, the minimal physical exertion in the form of a few steps in front of my apartment was enough to make my body sweat.

At this point I realized that I still had to take it easy, I had a long fever period behind me and had to accept that I would have to take it easy for a few more days or what it meant to me to rest. After some time tossing and turning in bed, I managed to sink into a restless sleep, and that night I was haunted by mysterious dreams that could best be compared to the kind of dreams you experience when you have a high fever. A significant difference, however, was that the dreams were accompanied by a dull and deep-seated feeling of anxiety that slowly built up and continued to increase until I suddenly woke up with palpitations and lay in my bed in panic, soaked in sweat.

The feeling of alienation that I felt when I tried to go for a walk had returned. I still remember clearly that this cycle of sleep, nightmares and the startled awakening was repeated several times that night until I woke up in the morning with a feeling as if a truck had hit me.

I sat absent-mindedly in the kitchen with my cup, wondering what had happened the day before and why I felt so exhausted. Because any feelings of alienation had disappeared, profound exhaustion spread through me, which I still find difficult to put into words today.

My cup of coffee seemed unnaturally heavy and sitting in the kitchen, which I found extremely comfortable, was tantamount to an effort. I smoked a cigarette and sank into my world of thoughts.

"Something's wrong with me," I murmured as I looked out of my kitchen window and felt the desire to leave my apartment to get some sun. With one last sip, I emptied my coffee cup and was reasonably motivated to go outside again for a walk.

"Everything will be normal again today," I said to myself as I took my keys and left my apartment. Outside I walked a few steps and crossed the road, my destination was about 300 meters away, where the buildings ended, and turned into a small forest that I had known since my childhood, because I have moved many times in my life, but have never left my hometown. I felt every step excruciatingly exhausting and felt a feeling of alienation rising in me again as if I was not properly connected to my body. Halfway along the way, my perception clouded and a kind of dizziness spread through me.

I fought my way forward for a few more meters but decided that it would be best if I turned back. I wanted to get back to my safe apartment quickly, as I felt incredibly vulnerable outside. At about the height of the parking spaces in front of the house, my neighbour approached me and engaged me in a superficial conversation, the content of which was as important as last year's dried shrubs in our flower boxes in front of the house. Although I never thought much of superficial small talk, I was always willing to exchange a few nice words, but after just a few sentences I had the feeling that I couldn't follow my neighbor's words anymore.

Each of her spoken words arrived in my head, but I couldn't stay focused. I just wanted to escape the situation. I explained to her in a few words that I had Covid and that I wasn't feeling very well.

"Not that you have Long Covid. I've heard something about it," she replied. With her words in mind, I went back to my apartment to rest.

The next few days went by and although my sleep was still not restful, some energy returned to my body. I drove my car to a field to do a lap across the field on foot. In retrospect, the first major flare-up of the disease occurred on that day. My mind was conditioned to the fact that I only had to try hard enough and everything would work, this may be true in many areas of life, after all, the lazy person rarely achieves his goals. Unfortunately, when it comes to health, false ambition can also produce the opposite effect. So I walked quickly along the edge of the field, actually, I liked this kind of walking very much, but everything felt like a burden.

"I have to go this round now and then I'll get fit again. I'll go through with it now, come what may."

I whipped myself forward and after a few hundred meters it was back, the feeling of alienation, which caused me great fear. My heart began to race and I squinted my eyes, the sun creating an unnatural brightness and burning on my skin. Although April was not hot, I felt as if I was crossing the North African desert, because I was also starting to find it difficult to breathe. At the end of the path, some field workers were in the process of setting up an irrigation system, and although I was already struggling with the worry that I might have a neurological failure, these people who could be my salvation scared me incredibly.

I know it may sound paradoxical, but I would not have been able to ask for help and draw attention to my situation, as an incredible fear flowed through my body. I fought my way back to my car and slumped exhausted in the driver's seat. My heart was pounding wildly. I folded down the sunshade to see the pale man with the reddened eyes again in the mirror inside.

I needed help, I knew that, I didn't want to go to the hospital because I was still scared. But I pulled my cell phone out of my pocket and made an appointment with my family doctor for the next day. I described that my sleep was disturbed, movement strained me unnaturally, I react strongly to light and stimuli and my pulse gets out of control, especially when I switch from sitting to a standing position.

My doctor showed understanding of my situation, but could not do much other than refer me to the cardiologist and extend my inability to work for fourteen days. After I left the practice, I picked up the phone and made a cardiological appointment in May. Somehow relieved (the specialist will get me back on track), I made an appointment with my best friend. Going for a walk together is better than alone.

I set off and drove a bit on the highway to pick up my friend at his apartment. I found the radio unbearable and had to concentrate on keeping my lane while driving.

"You look like shit in my face," my friend greeted me as I got in. We drove to a piece of forest where we wanted to hike. It helped me, even though symptoms came up again, my friend made me feel safe, so I was ready to go beyond my limits and we walked through the forest. When I got back home, my condition tipped over within a very short time, my heart began to race again and my consciousness clouded over. I took a shower to slow down a bit, but the water burned on my feet, which felt cold. I lost my balance and collapsed. I lay on the ground for a few minutes and gathered my strength.

I got dressed and knew that my next destination would be the hospital. I didn't know what was wrong with me, but I knew I desperately needed a doctor who could tell me. The car ride, which was not far, turned out to be a real adventure. With difficulty, I made it to the emergency room, where the first thing to do was to write an ECG, so far inconspicuous. Only my resting heart rate was 144 beats a minute.

"Go home and rest," said the attending physician. "I don't see any abnormalities on the ECG."

I felt misunderstood and rejected, but I didn't want to make a scene either, so I accepted the situation as it was and went back home.

The following days I rested and slowly recovered. I didn't feel healthy, but I was confident that things would finally go uphill. I also completed small training sessions and went small laps in front of the door. But I noticed that little by little the symptoms came back. They were latent all the time and whenever I felt better, they flared up more strongly. I didn't understand what kind of state I was in.

In the course of the next few weeks, events came thick and fast. The death of my grandmother is worth mentioning, as I reproached myself for a long time that I lacked the strength to be there for my family during this time and that I could not mourn her death because my health was bad.

On the day of the funeral, I felt like an empty shell that was completely occupied with itself and its symptoms and no longer could be in the here and now or even to mourn. My life consisted only of repetitive spirals of thoughts, worry about my condition, the fear of possible symptoms and the dwindling confidence in my own body.

I felt unspeakably exhausted and burned out after the funeral, spent the rest of my day in bed and finally fell asleep. In my dream, I was standing at a large floor-to-ceiling window, in a house unknown to me.

I looked through it and looked into a beautiful garden where flowers stood and large trees cast their shadows.

"I want to go there," I said in the dream.

"That's not possible, you're seriously ill, Christoph," someone answered.

I turned around and in front of me, I saw a reflection of myself. "You're sick, Christoph, very sick," it said in my voice.

I was startled out of this dream, sweat running down my chest, my body burning and the muscles in my thighs twitching. I collapsed, everything revolved around me, and my breathing was shallow and fast. I turned on the light in my bedroom and was overwhelmed. I could hardly stand on my feet, because my pulse seemed to get faster from moment to moment. I reached for my cell phone and without thinking twice, I dialled 112.

I dragged myself to the front door, it was about 5 a.m. I lay down on the cold steps until the ambulance arrived. On the way to the hospital, I seriously asked myself whether I could die, because this condition did not feel otherwise.

The paramedic, on the other hand, did not take me seriously, I reported severe pain and shortness of breath, but except for my pulse, which was again beyond 140, there were no abnormalities at first. In the hospital, I was back in the emergency room, in the same room where I had been diagnosed with the Covid infection a short time ago. This time, however, I had to keep my eyes closed, as the pattern of the ceiling and the sounds of the medical equipment were a complete sensory overload for me.

What followed was a marathon through the various fields of medicine, an ECG was followed by various blood tests, an X-ray of the lungs was taken and finally an ultrasound examination of the heart was performed. The doctor explained to me in detail what was in the picture, and despite my poor condition, I was happy that I was examined and felt understood.

"First of all, nothing to determine except tachycardia and a high inflammation level in the blood," the doctor spoke reassuringly. "You are suffering from a post-covid state," he continued. In the further conversation, he explained to me some theories from the medical side as to why this kind of consequence can occur, but basically, it is not clarified and so far only makes assumptions.

He cannot and will not be able to give me a recommendation. With the diagnosis in my luggage and back home, something began that I would describe today as one of my biggest mistakes and yet the best thing I could do: Googling. I spent countless hours researching and reading up on a wide variety of medical conditions. I only left my apartment when necessary, the experience had frightened me for a long time and took the courage to try again. I took it easy as best I could, but no matter how little I did, the palpitations didn't seem to go away, a change of position in bed was enough to get my pulse going.

When I got up, it got worse, when I showered, I noticed that my legs were marbling and turning blue. Since I knew my symptoms by now, I started looking for answers on the Internet, and finally, I stopped at a disease with the abbreviated name POTS.

Armed with my assumption, I wandered through the city centre somewhat disoriented, my cardiologist appointment was due, and although I had known the city since I was born and had a good sense of direction, I wandered through the alleys and only managed to find the practice with the help of passers-by whom I approached. I reported in detail and was then subjected to a kind of test in which you move from the sitting position to the standing position while blood pressure and pulse are measured. In fact, after this test, I collected the next diagnosis of POTS.

In addition, heart failure was suspected (which, thank God, did not come true), but for the moment I was provided with pills. Especially the drainage tablets bothered me. Since my COVID-19 infection, I have been dehydrated many times and water that I drank glided through me without resistance and the antihypertensive drugs also made my situation worse.

I am grateful that I was able to stop taking the medication very quickly, as a blood test revealed that I did not suffer from heart failure. Against the tachycardia syndrome, I should start cycling, maybe you have affected yourself and can imagine what happened now: The total fall into the abyss. My parents owned a small bicycle, with which I would try to do a short lap three times a week from now on. The first few times worked out well, I rode a kilometre and had the feeling that I could now actively do something to get healthy.

But when I set off on my second lap a few days later, I found that I only managed a third of my first distance. It went on like this over 14 days, my symptoms continued to increase in intensity and the long-term ECG I had to wear stressed me immensely. I wanted to be healthy, I was always healthy and decided that I just had to try a lot harder. I phoned doctors twice, my health insurance company offered a corresponding service.

On the first phone call, I spoke to an internist who encouraged me, and the second time I was connected to a cardiologist who, after I had described my symptoms to him, advised me to read up on a help page for CFS. He used terms that I couldn't classify, such as pacing, but I didn't follow his advice for the time being and thought I'd get a grip on it again, even if everything was getting worse instead of better. I got eye drops at the pharmacy and tried to do something good for myself with intestinal bacteria. Further healing attempts with natural blood thinners and all conceivable herbs followed, which were freely available for sale, I experimented around like a headless chicken and spent a lot of money. At that time, it was still small amounts. But in the course of my story, they will add up to an amount of over 20,000 euros, which I spent unsuccessfully in the hope of a cure.

At that time, I also noticed that I was isolating myself more and more, when I lent the bike from my parents, I often did it when no one was home. I love my parents and today I love spending time with them, but back then, when I got sick, I avoided people out of shame about my condition or to avoid making them sad by seeing how bad I was.

I also cancelled other important appointments, such as the treatment of my teeth, I just couldn't manage to go to the doctor and get treatment. Just the thought of lying at the dentist overwhelmed me. I'm not an anxious patient, because I've spent a lot of my life with dentists – I've been through everything from root tip resection to tooth extraction, but I wasn't physically and mentally able to get treatment. Everything that had nothing to do with my condition receded into the background. The only person I had allowed to get close to me was my girlfriend. I texted her by cell phone that I would now go for a long ride on my bike. I drove off and fought against the physical weakness, I drove on and on along the streets and it got worse and worse.

I don't know how I got home from my parents after the bike ride, my memory is more than clouded. I stumbled into my apartment, everything was spinning, and my pulse broke through the 200 mark. I measured my blood pressure 211 to 122.

I fell on the sofa and lost consciousness. When I came to, my body was pulsating and yet I was paralyzed. I wanted to get help, but my phone seemed unreachable. I had lost all strength to move. Renewed unconsciousness. I came to, it had become dark outside, I realized that I had been lying here for hours, and I still lacked the strength to get up. I lay there in incredible pain, everything hurt from my foot to my head and since I was no longer able to do anything, I asked myself if I was going to die.

I am aware that this sounds extremely dramatic, but at that moment I began to come to terms with my life. In total, I lay on my sofa in this state for about 48 hours, unable to speak in my sweat and severe physical pain. At some point, this condition subsided a bit, so I managed to get from the sofa to bed, where I lay awake until the next morning. Overall, I lay for a period of three to four days in which I didn't eat anything or sleep.

My phone rang, but I was blocked. I couldn't lose weight. Speaking simple words seemed to be an indescribable effort, clear thoughts were no longer possible. My head was in a deep fog, my body was failing. When some energy returned after some time, I managed to walk around my apartment and make myself a sandwich. I recovered physically, but from now on I spent most of my day in bed, I was a broken man.

During this time, my girlfriend took care of me, I was not able to take care of anything, even a phone call overwhelmed me. Shopping had become an impossibility, I could only shower while sitting and I had to force the one slice of bread I ate a day. In general, I noticed that eating worsened my condition, I reacted with palpitations and severe exhaustion when I tried to eat a little more.

I lost 14 kilos of weight during this time, and even though my girlfriend always tried to get me to eat, I just couldn't do it. I now spend my time on the Internet, I joined some Long Covid groups and exchanged ideas with other sufferers. I had arrived in the valley of tears, please don't get me wrong, I know from my own experience what it's like to be so sick, but basically, many of the groups were a gathering place for stranded people who compete to see who is more severely affected or spread the word that no one will recover and that we are all lost. I was quickly made aware that my situation sounds like the disease ME/CFS. I studied the Internet and was shocked to find that some self-help groups predicted an incredibly agonizing death for me, dramatized, and many of those affected also told me that there would be no cure.

In the next few days, I fell into a state of grief and shock, I was a sporty man, just over 30 years old, how could my life be over now?

Would I now be plagued by these symptoms for the rest of my life? I was mentally at my wit's end. I remember lying in bed crying with a panic attack, begging my girlfriend to help me.

"Someone has to help me, please, I need help!"

I cried and cried for help, never did I feel more powerless in my life. This memory still gives me a queasy feeling today, because it symbolizes the absolute low point of my life. Even though I am averse to Long Covid groups on social media today, I got to know a few people who accompanied me on my way. One of these people was called Martin, a father of two and himself severely affected and almost mostly confined to his bed. We exchanged ideas every day, which didn't make me feel any better, but I had found a person who was in the same boat, and although Martin was even more affected than I was, he always encouraged me.

We both agreed that no matter how bad we are and how desperate we are, we will get well again. One day we were talking about blood washes because at that time there were the first reports on YouTube. I joined a group on Facebook that dealt with the topic of immune absorption antibodies being washed out of the blood that runs through a filter. Nobody knew whether this type of treatment would bring anything for Long Covid, as testimonials were still rare and they ranged from at least temporary improvements to deteriorations. I was desperate enough to grasp at every straw, I was so sick by now that I was just lying in bed and every activation attempt failed. The private medical treatment in which I found myself in the meantime did not help me. I only bought expensive dietary supplements, which of course didn't help at all and the specialist mostly shrugged my shoulders. There was no therapy. So I paid the private doctor to take my blood and have it tested for autoantibodies and after a week I got the result: out of seven possible categories, I fulfilled six.

I felt as if I had found the solution and wrote to all university hospitals to carry out such an absorption on me. Since I only received rejections or my e-mail was not answered, I looked for a private provider and found it in Hanover. I would have to pay 15,000 euros for hotel and treatment, although the outcome was completely unclear, I didn't hesitate for a minute. At that moment it seemed like the chance to save my life and whoever is desperate and owns a nail suddenly sees a hammer in everything.

Martin also set his appointments in August 2022, so we would leave for Hanover at the same time. Every day we wrote and were extremely excited, we encouraged each other and that we would soon be healthy.

In retrospect, we did something during this time that would later be relevant to my recovery, we visualized health. Since we were both extremely sensitive to temperatures and the summer was already extremely warm, Martin decided to postpone his appointments to September, and he suffered a severe breakdown when he tried to shower one day.

It happened that I didn't hear from Martin for several days because he was too bad to listen to voice messages or write anything, but whenever he felt better, he got in touch with me again. Every morning he sent me a screenshot of a calendar where a day was crossed off and supported me immensely, even if we are no longer in contact today, I am grateful to him from the bottom of my heart.

I spent my time at home and my social contacts were limited to my girlfriend and some contacts that I maintained online. I was grateful to my girlfriend for getting through this time with me, as

I woke her up several times almost every night as my sleep disorders were at their peak. I lay awake most of the time and dealt with my symptoms until I slipped into a light sleep. This was usually characterized by bad nightmares, which often had biographical references.

I could hardly bear touch at that time, mostly we slept back to back because everything beyond that was too much for me. This situation was unbearable, I felt physically, mentally and emotionally crippled, and I wanted nothing more than to regain my health, but in the end, I was a prisoner in my own body, haunted by over 50 different symptoms.

I was ready to go into the unknown, I had nothing left to lose, as I thought I would spend the rest of my life in my apartment to slowly go to the dogs. My girlfriend booked me a hotel and my brother agreed to go with me to Hanover, he would stay there for the first night, but then have to return home. I knew that I would be taken care of at the hotel (there was one breakfast a day, which was sufficient because I hardly ate any food) and the 300 meters that had to be covered to the place of treatment, I would take a taxi.

Even though the private doctor advised me against the treatment at that time, as its outcome was not predictable, I put all my hopes in it. Since I had written to all university hospitals in North Rhine-Westphalia without success (from today's point of view, of course, I understand these rejections, basically someone contacted me by e-mail claiming that he had Long Covid and asked for a treatment for which there were not even studies, but I was desperate and tried, no matter how unlikely an answer was from today's point of view), I knew, that I would have to take everything into my own hands.

I often felt as if my time was running out, not in the sense that a deadly disease would take me away, but my greatest fear was chronification. In the groups, there was a lot of talk about Canadian criteria and times and this set in my head that I would be lost after half a year in which the disease would exist. From my point of view today, I know that this is not true, but only a diagnostic criterion, but in my situation at that time I hung up on it.

You were sick and had the whole day to look for answers on the Internet and compare your symptoms with different clinical pictures, it was terrible behaviour that did more harm, but there was no one there who could say: "Relax, Christoph, on day XY you will be healthy again and everything will be fine, lean back."

I had the private doctor test me for glandular fever, as this could probably be reactivated by Covid and this test was an important prerequisite for immunoadsorption. I wouldn't have been surprised if it had been positive, at least I would have had an explanation why I always felt like I was getting a bad flu.

My immune system felt like it was permanently activated and I often suffered lymph node swelling. The doctor tested me and ruled out a lot, I had no cancer, no diabetes, no depression and no reactive EBV. She prescribed me antihistamines to get my reaction to food under control, I also took them for a while but then stopped taking them again.

My diet currently consists only of oatmeal and rice. I had now made all the preparations and packed my bag with clothes that my girlfriend had ordered for me, as I was not able to go shopping and wrote a lot with Martin that evening.

He encouraged me that I would now go to Hanover and fight for my health, I would be strong and would get everything over with without any problems. He would try to become more stable as quickly as possible and then leave as soon as he could. Martin's words did me good, he was almost a kind of big brother to me in this situation. He turned a lot to religion during this time and tried to get the time as best he could. While I was still able to walk around my apartment a bit, he was just lying in bed, he often didn't even manage to sit.

Chapter 3
A trip to Hanover with

earplugs and sunglasses

At the end of July 2022, the time had come, in the morning Martin sent me a calendar on which today was circled, and it finally started. I had great respect for the trip, on this day the temperatures cracked the 30-degree Celsius mark and we left in the morning. With sunglasses and noise protection, I lay down on the back seat with a pillow, where I tried to perceive as few external stimuli as possible.

We hardly talked during the trip. I occasionally opened my eyes and saw trucks that we were overtaking. Everything felt surreal, what had happened? A few months ago I was still healthy and now I was lying in the back seat of a car that drove me to a foreign city for medical treatment with an unclear outcome.

My thoughts were circling, actually I didn't know how I was going to get along alone in Hanover, there was a possibility that my girlfriend or my mother would have accompanied me, but I didn't want that, after all, I also reckoned with the risk that I would not tolerate the treatment and since I couldn't imagine how bad it would have been for me in that case, I didn't want to have anyone around me whom I would have burdened with it.

When I arrived at the hotel, my brother spoke to the ladies at the reception described my situation and asked them to bring breakfast to my room and to check on me in general as soon as he had left. I used the day of arrival to rest as best as possible and to pursue my only hobby, internet research.

For weeks, I had been combing through hundreds of websites, reading studies and researching on the way to finding a solution. I joined various forums and found myself in several Facebook groups. In retrospect, I lost myself here and slipped into a parallel world in which I dealt exclusively with diseases, only to be left with more questions than answers in the end.

After a night in which I slept for a few hours, my brother took me to the treatment rooms in the morning. I was ushered into a room in which there were six beds, three on each side of the wall, and beside them were large white machines to which were attached an innumerable number of tubes that directed the blood into a filter.

I was weighed, and the scales showed a weight of 80 kilograms on its digital display, I had lost 14 kilos, but I didn't care. I was now here to be treated and maybe even cured, and after a blood pressure measurement (this was 200 to 105) it finally started. I was given two entrances by a doctor so that the blood could flow from my right arm into the machine, and then returned to my body washed via my left arm, while everything was accompanied by a cracking sound of the machine.

On the day of my first treatment, I lay in my treatment bed for almost seven hours and kept my eyes mostly closed, my sunglasses protected me from the bright light in the room and my noise protectors somewhat dampened the hustle and bustle of the hospital around me. While nurses and doctors were busy in the room, changing bags, laying accesses or doing other work, I withdrew into my world of thoughts. My gaze often wandered out of the window for a few seconds, through which you could see a park, I remembered a dream I had at the beginning of my illness. Outside was a green area with many trees casting their shadows. I imagined going out there and enjoying the summer, and then there it was, the voice from my dream: "No, Christoph, that's not possible, you're seriously ill."

I looked around the room and watched the tubes through which my blood flowed and said quietly to myself, "Yes, I am." A tear flowed under my sunglasses. The next day I completed the second treatment, followed by a few days of rest, as the six applications would take place over 21 days. I experienced an up and down of emotions. On the one hand, I was strengthened by the feeling that I was doing something for my health here, but on the other hand, I was very afraid and tense.

At that time, I made a statement that I saw as a direct consequence of the treatment at the time but would be repeated again and again in my later vacations. I felt better physically. Between the third and fourth blood washes, I developed conjunctivitis and was so emotionally battered that I lay crying on the floor of the hotel at night, feeling indescribably alone. I didn't want to be here in this strange city, with these strange people and be connected to this strange machine.

The next day, however, I plucked up the courage to go to the REWE store, it was paradoxical, a few hours ago I had experienced a mental breakdown and now I was on my way to the supermarket on foot. It was an incredibly beautiful experience, I saw people walking through the market and doing their shopping, it was the first everyday scene I witnessed after months of isolation.

I felt torn away from my parallel world for a moment and although I was incredibly weak, I enjoyed being in the world of the healthy. Taking new courage that recovery would certainly come soon, I even talked to patients who were lying in the beds next to me during the upcoming treatments. Everyone here was affected in some way and fought against long-term effects.

I was one of the more severely affected, but some people were far worse off than I was. A gratitude that was difficult to describe rose in me. Although I was only a shadow of myself at the time, I felt gratitude for being able to wash myself or make myself a coffee.

I remembered my first big breakdown, in which brushing my teeth was a real feat of strength and fatigue crushed me so much that talking was too exhausting. I could hardly do anything now, but more than then. For the first time, I developed a kind of acceptance for my situation and was confident that a turning point would come. I decided to return here in the fall, as a healthy man, to visit Ahmed during his treatment. I imagined what it would be like to come here healthy and imagined it down to the smallest detail.

The last two treatments passed without any incidents worth mentioning, I was happy to say goodbye to Hanover and to have survived everything in one piece. My brother noticed positive changes in me very quickly, I seemed more alert and spoke more than on the way there. At the height of Wuppertal, I even sat upright for a while and watched the passing highway for a while.

I was looking forward to going home, I had made it. When I got home, I fell into a deep state of exhaustion, which lasted for the next 14 days, as I was supposed to isolate myself until my immune system was fully capable of acting again, I spent the time alone and wrote a first experience report in the Facebook group about immune absorptions.

At that time, the groups were still an important part of my life, but I knew that as soon as I got better, I would trade the groups for my friends and family. The days went by and my exhaustion improved slightly, I waited eagerly for the moment when everything would disappear, I imagined myself waking up in the morning and feeling normal, but I waited in vain.

I clung to the hope that it was only a matter of time, person X said it would take six weeks, and person Y claimed that it could be twelve before noticeable effects would occur. I was confused and disappointed, somehow I felt slightly better, and in Hanover, I was even able to do a little shopping, but here at home, I was exhausted again and waited in vain for my healing.

Although there was no guarantee that the treatment would have a positive effect, I clung to it so much, after all, it was the only thing I could do from my knowledge at the time. What other options were open to me? Rest did not bring me any relief, a miracle drug did not exist and other offers from the medical side consisted of rehab. But I knew that I would never do it. I was an athlete and had been for almost twenty years if a few push-ups had been the way to freedom, I would have been healthy three times, but exercise was not a big option for me and put a lot of strain on me when I tried.

In addition, on the one hand, you were always confronted with the fact that there were no studies to make a well-founded statement about my condition, but on the other hand I was offered rehab, but there were no studies of it either, that didn't fit together for me. If I had suffered a car accident or had to overcome a physical limitation for some other reason, I would have gone to rehab with a waving flag, but I just had the feeling that they wanted to treat a diabetic with sugar.

Chapter 4
Relapse but new hope

As the weeks went by, I became increasingly frustrated and sad. I asked myself many questions, what did the bloodwashing do for me? Why did I feel better in Hanover? Do autoantibodies have an influence, and can I get healthy at all? I spent hours pondering. My days were minimally more active than before, which meant that I only lay 20 hours a day and I sometimes dared to go to the mailbox, or I tried to keep in touch with friends and family, but the symptoms were still my constant companion.

While I appreciated this kind of improvement, I felt like I was treading water or going around in circles, on top of that, my friend Richard was also complaining of a slight deterioration after his immune absorption at the time, and I couldn't find answers in ME/CFS or Long Covid groups, but often ran into embittered people, who had long since left the topic of healing behind.

From my current point of view, I cannot conclusively judge what influence the treatment had on my path to healing, I experienced an improvement that unfortunately regressed, but cognitively I reached a point that allowed me to think more clearly. My friend Richard sent me the link to an American YouTube channel one morning. Although I was only able to follow the videos for a maximum of ten minutes at a time, I consumed them as often as I could.

The channel was run by a woman who had suffered from CFS herself for ten years and conducted interviews with people who had also overcome the disease.

In the beginning, I was very skeptical, on my way so far I have often been confronted with alleged healings. However, I quickly realized that no one wanted to sell me anything on this channel, but people simply told their stories. I was confronted with many new views and was amazed at how many people had managed to leave this state behind and are now living a normal life again. I watched dozens of the videos over a long period and began to deal with recovery stories in general, to the point where I realized for myself that all these people were telling the truth, while in German-speaking forums I was almost religiously persuaded that getting well is not possible.

I decided to leave all forums and groups behind me and end all contact except with Martin and Richard. I was tired of being in this toxic environment that confronted me every day with how bad everyone was. Please don't get me wrong, but I believe that distancing yourself from negatively minded people is almost a kind of basic prerequisite for one's recovery.

Likewise, I decided to stop any internet search that didn't address recovery. I didn't care what Dr. So-Anyway found out, or what Charité wrote, it just triggered me and any articles that drug XYZ will soon go into research had become completely irrelevant to me. I decided to make my cure a top priority and after all the failed attempts at medication, various natural remedies and immune absorption, I was ready to throw everything overboard and start over.

I also discovered a German YouTube channel of a victim who gave me many valuable tips. I got to know the different theories of the disease and the role of the nervous system in them, I was aware that much was not scientifically proven, but it sounded more than conclusive to me. As a pragmatic person, I said goodbye to the idea that my immune system had a defect and stopped looking to doctors for an answer.

At this point, I would like to mention that I do not deny any physician his competence and that I always confidently seek medical treatment when necessary, but in my situation, there were no answers, and until medicine can provide them, years of research could still take place. I tore myself away from everything that had gone before to find my answers. I began to think a lot about my life, and during this time I experienced strong biographical dreams when I slept. I reflected on the last few years and realized that I was suffering from symptoms long before the actual onset of my illness as if a subconscious voice had tried to draw my attention to the fact that something was wrong with my lifestyle years ago.

At this point I realized for the first time how aimless and unhappy I had been in life, I always had one goal and that was money, but realized that I wanted to get this money primarily to plug holes in my soul. I did everything to achieve this goal, I sacrificed my health for it, except for a few moral boundaries, I didn't care about anything, I was ready to use any means to reach my goal. I only realized that I would be the loser in the end at that time when I thought about my life for the first time.

I recognized the connection: Before my illness, I was always rushing around to fix problems, but I never solved my problems in the long term, I usually hastily poured a bucket of water on the flames and then moved to the next source of fire, without noticing that the embers were still there and that the same fire would soon break out again. With Long Covid I behaved similarly, I rushed around and tried everything without achieving success and that stressed me out immensely, it was the water on the millstone that kept my symptoms going.

I started meditating and it was terrible, a resistance to let go built up in me, as if my brain was saying: "We are in mortal danger! How can you think about relaxation now? We have to be vigilant!"

I began to tremble, my body trying to slide into relaxation, but at the same time, it seemed to block itself, as if you were trying to sleep, even though you knew that a fire was about to break out. I used a trick that I had learned from Richard, he was reading a book that dealt with neurogenic tremors, which can occur after shock, for example. So before my next attempt at meditation, I lay on my back and lifted my pelvis and in fact, I produced the same tremor as when I first tried to meditate.

I was amazed and confirmed that my body was actually trying to find rest, but first, the tension (by the way, it was so great that I lost 3.5 mm of my teeth due to grinding) had to tremble away. I didn't use the technique for long, over a maximum period of two months, but it helped me a lot, especially in the beginning. Now that I was able to bring my body down a bit, I learned to meditate and tried to clear my head of the worries and thoughts of illness that constantly plagued me.

All beginnings are hard and it sounded easier said than done when you can only walk 300 to 400 steps a day and otherwise only look at your wall, it's hard not to worry, but I did my best.

I got myself a piece of paper and began to write down what I could:

- Watch videos
- Go to the mailbox
- Shower
- Make me something to eat
- Meditate

I was a bit sad that my life had shrunk to this manageable number of activities, but I was very confident that I would soon be able to extend the list. As the year 2022 was slowly coming to an end, my first big goal was to celebrate Christmas together with my parents or at least eat with them for an hour. I also achieved this goal, I enjoyed being united with my family very much, even though I noticed after a short time that four people overwhelmed my capacities. My head closed at one point and the dizziness set in.

My girlfriend drove me home, and even though I was done, I was happy to have achieved this goal. Richard also spent the party with his family in northern Germany, we exchanged ideas and celebrated our success. A violent flare-up of all symptoms followed,

I had gone beyond my limits and my thoughts slipped back into the world of fear and illness, I tried as best I could to relax my nervous system with meditations and distract myself from the negative thoughts.

Distraction was not easy as I didn't have many activities to fill my day, I was very limited in my scope of action but decided to find a new activity that I could tolerate. I hadn't touched a computer game for many years but decided to play the game Minetest, which you could download for free. It was just right for me, it didn't cause any stress, there were no enemies and no fights (it may sound weird, but light excitement was already too much for me at times) and in creative mode, I could just walk around the world and implement building projects.

I now played for half an hour a day and listened to recovery stories, and in fact, I managed to enjoy my playing time more and more and was able to switch off my thoughts. Whenever I noticed that it was getting too much for me, I would end the game and lie down to meditate. I tried to increase the amount of time I could work on the PC, of course, I was only playing one game, but I had started building a lighthouse and felt committed to the project. The difference between keeping an accounting department on the computer or playfully following a project is not as big as you think when you commit to treating your project like real work.

I kept increasing my time on the PC over the weeks and noticed that it tied up a lot of my capacities, but at the same time, I noticed further cognitive progress. I still suffered from brain fog, but I was able to concentrate longer and planned to build a harbour next to the lighthouse. So my time passed until January 2023, when I decided that I wanted to meet up with a friend. I tried to explain my situation to my friend Mark as well as possible and that it could happen that I had to end our appointment after ten minutes. I felt shame in the little world that I created for myself at home, I was reasonably safe, but when I made contact with healthy people, I often felt in need of an explanation and at the same time feared that I would not be understood.

Mark came up to me and we talked over a cup of coffee, I was very excited about the situation and imagined that my symptoms would get stronger at any moment, and that's what happened. I ended the appointment and lay down, my body pulsating and the muscles of my legs twitching violently. I felt in danger and my heart began to race. I knew I couldn't stop the symptoms, but my reaction to them shouldn't end in panic any further.

It took me a few days to recover, and then I looked into techniques to calm the nervous system and came across various breathing exercises that can activate the parasympathetic nervous system. The first became a kind of all-rounder for me, which I could use in between during the day or at night when I suffered from bad states of restlessness. It consisted of inhaling for four seconds, then holding your breath for another six seconds, and then exhaling slowly for about eight seconds.

After a few repetitions, I already noticed how I became noticeably calmer. The second exercise I learned was a stimulation of the vagus nerve, which involves humming while exhaling, precisely with the letters A U M, because the vibrations that are generated stimulate the nerve positively. This technique took longer to produce a noticeable effect, but it could be combined well with longer meditations. In addition, I acquired other relaxation exercises, my kit now consisted of:

- Meditation
- Breathing
- Neurogenic tremors
- Gargling (also stimulates the vagus nerve)
- Yawn
- Neck relaxation

- Cold showers

With these exercises, I now had the opportunity to do things for myself that were good for me, especially the cold shower proved to be a kind of secret weapon for me. Warm water still boosted my heart rate and put a strain on my circulation, but cold showers (I only took cold showers up to the height of my hips) had the opposite effect on me. It felt like my legs were being pulled together by the cold and the excess blood was being pushed back up.

Due to the POTS, everything felt like it slid down, if I stood too long, my feet turned blue and my legs formed a spotted pattern. We were still in January 2023, but the coming summer was already worrying me, as my temperature regulation felt like it was failing at anything above 20 degrees. I sweat profusely, but the opportunity to take cold showers gave me courage. I didn't feel so exposed and helpless anymore.

During this time I slept a lot, my sleep was still light and not restful, but I now took a nap almost every day and that did me a lot of good. It was a kind of constant structure that I usually fell asleep around 4 p.m. for an hour or two. Afterwards, I was often completely exhausted, but my body signalled to me a higher need for sleep, which I pursued.

February had come and with it new insights. Richard read up on a wide variety of topics and always shared his findings with me. He told me about the technique of visualization and that the brain would not necessarily distinguish between the world of thoughts and reality. He was currently reading a book on neuronal plasticity. To put it simply, it was about brain areas being able to restructure and adapt, Richard would tell me more in the coming weeks when he had read the book.

I arranged to meet Mark again, but this time at his home, I had plucked up the courage to leave my apartment. The appointment was short and exhausting, since Mark had moved into a new apartment that I didn't know yet, I felt insecure. Foreign places scared me and after about 15 minutes, when Mark told me that I was pale, I wanted to go home again.

A few days of severe symptoms followed, but then we met again at his place. I was surprised to find that the feeling of insecurity was still strong, but nowhere near as overwhelming as it had been on my first visit a few days earlier. I spent about half an hour with him before the brain fog became so strong that I had to go home. I had developed severe symptoms again after the meeting and lay in bed for a few days with a mixture of flu, anxiety and muscle twitches; but I knew that I would meet with Mark again to find out if it was a coincidence or if I could stay longer from time to time.

Since my girlfriend was often with me, and I now met Mark once a week, I felt like I had some kind of social life again and that made me happy. The following Friday I felt good by my standards, I had some energy and my girlfriend would come to spend the weekend with me. I decided to go with her to Schieß-bahn, a small neighbouring town that we often visited for walks before my illness.

A lap on the field was physically out of the question, but I wanted to stroll a little through the small city centre. Since my girlfriend understood me and always supported me, I wasn't afraid if I told her that we had to go, she understood, and it took a lot of pressure off me. For February it was warm on this day and so it happened that we walked a short distance and then sat down in an ice cream parlor.

I was overwhelmed with happiness. For the past nine months, I had been dreaming of this moment when I was eating ice cream with my girlfriend. The whole thing was exhausting, as I felt like a foreign body in the world of the healthy, but I had found a way for myself to regulate the emerging tensions a bit. After about ten minutes, I noticed that I was overwhelmed by the many people around us who were talking (actually the situation wasn't particularly loud, but I still reacted strongly to noises), so I retreated to the toilet of the ice cream parlour.

I locked myself in the cabin and thought about a place where I felt safe. I tried to slow down my breathing a bit and started with the four six eight breathing, while I talked to myself in my mind and kept repeating that I was safe in this place. The symptoms didn't go away, but I didn't panic either and managed to stay in the ice cream parlour for some time until we left home, where I fell exhausted on the bed.

I was exhausted and my body became heavy as lead, exhaustion struck with full force. At this point in my journey, breaks did not give me any rest, so I lay in bed as if paralyzed, staring at the wall. As so often, I had gone beyond my limits and lay awake at night, because I was so excited inside, strange people, a strange place and a lot of noises, that had taken a toll on me. But I had deliberately gone beyond my limits and from my research I knew that recovery would not be possible at all without a crash, so my long-term goal was to lose the fear of them. That was easier said than done and until I managed to finally let go of this fear, almost a year would pass because at the moment these breakdowns were still overwhelming.

I must have experienced over a hundred such breakdowns during my recovery because at first, only tolerance grows. When I was very sick, brushing my teeth was enough to make me crash, then it was going to the mailbox, then shopping and so on. This continued until my eventual recovery and the variations of these conditions were almost unlimited, for example, I experienced:

- Severe pain conditions with jaw and leg pain
- A strong feeling of illness accompanied by nerve pain
- Migraine-like conditions

- Biographical, bizarre dreams
- Sweating and circulatory disorders
- Vision problems and severe tinnitus
- Nausea and digestive problems
- countless other combinations

The symptoms were always accompanied by dizziness, and brain fog, and the insomnia always intensified extremely. So a few days passed until I had recovered and I was incredibly proud of myself for having made it this far.

Over the next few weeks, I met with Mark regularly and the meetups got better and better and slowly I got a feel for where my physical limits were. Richard, who had read the book on neuronal plasticity in the meantime, now provided me with new information every day, which further strengthened me. Since the brain is capable of learning, it should be possible to teach the brain that it does not have to produce these symptoms, as there is no reason for it.

Every step beyond the actual physical or emotional limits started the vicious circle and for us, the answer was to convince the brain that we were safe. We started to see a crash only as a kind of neurofeedback of the nervous system, even if the scientific explanation for Long Covid and CFS could be completely different or much more complex, this was still not important to us.

Many people have already become healthy and we could too. I focused on people who were further along in health than me or on those who had already recovered, to get as much information and context as possible. At the same time, I broke off contact with severely affected people, except for negative things or the plans for some drug treatments, I had nothing constructive to expect. When I felt steady better in the next few weeks (I increased to over 1000 steps a day, my maximum physical performance was about 3500 steps on very good days), I unfortunately lost contact with Martin at that time, I didn't want to break it off, but I think it hurt him a lot, that I was making progress while he was bedridden, which I could understand. I wish him all the best from the bottom of my heart and that he regains his health.

With my increasing health, I tried to participate in normal life again, I sometimes arranged to meet my mother to go for a short walk with the dogs or took on the responsibility of looking after the dogs when my parents had to work. The job was easy and not strenuous, but it gave me the feeling that I was accomplishing something and had fixed appointments again.

My brother also stopped by regularly while I looked after the dogs, and we usually sat together for a coffee and talked. My grandfather, who was very worried about me, also started cooking for me every day. After the loss of his wife and my illness, we spent an hour of the day together every day for months and thus bridged the loneliness that burdened both of us.

Richard made huge leaps at that time and surpassed me physically (I believe that every recovery is individual and while my cognitive abilities returned first and the physical ones were a long time coming, he went blow after blow). He started regular walks again spent a lot of time in nature and engaged in new activities such as mushroom picking.

I was very happy for him and even though I didn't trust myself to go for walks yet, I was in good spirits that I would soon be able to do it again. But as of now, physical exertion would still be fatal for me, so I thought about how I could continue and planned that in the evening if I could, I would walk a few meters along the edge of the field, even if the thought made me a little insecure. At the beginning of the disease, I often tried to force myself to walk, putting myself in a worse and worse situation. So I meditated for a few days and kept imagining how I would go for a walk and not get any symptoms. I dared my first attempt in the dark and walked a little up the dirt road, the lanterns seemed to shine unnaturally brightly so that I had to squint my eyes a bit. I managed about 150 meters until I realized that it was now time to turn back. The next few weeks I went the same way again and again and laboriously worked my way on, usually I managed to go one lantern further than the previous week. But sometimes I also took steps backwards and achieved less. The trick was not to react frustrated.

I often thought that I could set goals that I would achieve in certain periods. For example, I said that in the summer I would be at 100 per cent, even though I was aware that it wouldn't be like that. On the one hand, it was disappointing because I was never able to reach my time targets, but on the other hand, I created a self-fulfilling prophecy.

My conviction that the nervous system was responsible for all this became more and more firmly established in me, nerves and immune systems were out of control, and to heal, they would have to be brought back to a normal state. I also came across some American doctors, some of them neurologists, who held the same view. I didn't need direct scientific proof, because for me it was the most meaningful thesis I've heard so far.

If we are honest, if I had not achieved success, I would probably have rejected it again, but I felt the real improvement in my own body. I tried to convince those affected by this theory but often found that the interest was usually non-existent. But it wasn't important to me either, health is something highly personal and I had neither the right nor was it not my task to proselytize. I preferred to talk to people who had managed to recover, there were some of them, but they were difficult to grasp.

I could understand it too, if I had my life back, I wouldn't waste my precious time being present on the internet telling everyone my story. But also a neurologist, to whom I went at the request of my doctor, told me that the prognosis of post-virally acquired CFS does not always have to be so bad. From his experience, people who have recovered withdraw completely and go about their lives while others stay behind, so there is also the impression that no one will get better.

I decided to enjoy my life as much as I could and to carry on as before. I had a slight upward trend, so my path could not be wrong, even if I was often plagued by doubts about it. The fear that I wouldn't recover played a very big role. I was worried that I would end up in a wheelchair and no longer be able to take care of myself. I was afraid of being forgotten and of being all alone in the end – disappeared from society.

Even though I actively fought these thoughts, they always hovered over me like a sword of Damocles, this fixation on my condition also improved gradually, but was sometimes more stressful than some physical symptoms. I was never a person who liked to talk about my worries or fears, but slowly learned that it is not a weakness to communicate them openly. When the fear of the disease overwhelmed me, I shared it with my friend, who always showed me full understanding and built me up mentally.

She always reminded me of the progress I had already made and encouraged me, I felt understood and not alone and usually the anxious mood subsided after just one day and then disappeared.

Chapter 5
An arduous path to the top

Spring had come and with it further progress. In the last few weeks, I always took two steps forward and one step back, sometimes it was three steps back, but deterioration was temporary and usually limited to a few days. In the meantime, I was able to watch entire films again, and while I was watching a film with my girlfriend, I thought about how I visited my mother shortly after my trip to Hanover.

I watched a documentary about Lapland with her, which looked something like this: I always watched the film for a few minutes and then closed my eyes again because it was too much of a strain on me. But now I watched the movie with pleasure and only realized towards the end that I needed a break.

In general, my progress was noticeable on every level, some of my symptoms such as tinnitus and sensitivity to light slowly dissolved and others such as the jaw grinding or the vibration of my body decreased significantly, it felt like there was less pressure on the kettle. What still bothered me badly were the sleep disorders, after I slept for a maximum of five hours at a time for the first ten months, there was also a slight progression here (sometimes I managed six hours), but I finally wanted to be able to sleep normally again.

I tried a lot, but at the beginning, nothing worked, no sleeping tea, no herbs and no melatonin, but since I was now feeling better overall, I wanted to give the latter another chance. I got some in my pharmacy and found out that same evening that it had a good effect on me, for the coming months it would become a permanent companion for me.

In April, almost exactly one year after my infection, I became infected with Covid again, the fear was great and the uncertainty as to whether everything was in vain and I would end up in a wheelchair after all. I realized that everything that had happened was trauma to me, and the mere thought of it terrified me. But I had no choice. The infection was there and started with a fever like the first time, but far milder and my brain fog, which returned during the infection, was also weaker.

After a week I was negative again and knew exactly what I had to do now, I had to keep my feet still and give my body the space to recover. For a fortnight I experienced a deterioration in my condition, especially the palpitations and the physical weakness increased again, but my way of dealing with it was now different. I accepted it, and for the first time in my life, I was ready to accept that my body is not a machine that has to obey me and that you simply have to take it easy after a viral infection.

I used the time at home and meditated a lot and dealt with many things that I ran away from for years. Slowly, a picture began to emerge for me as to why the disease had come into my life in the first place. I always pushed myself to the extreme and the overexploitation of my body was normal for me. I lived a life with extremes, whether it was sports or work, I never knew a healthy mediocrity. Fortunately, I was never an alcoholic, but when I drank, there was no stopping me there either. Usually, I didn't return home until the morning hours, so drunk that I couldn't pronounce my name.

Beer wasn't enough, it had to be schnapps. I behaved similarly in business, I can say that I never harmed anyone out of bad faith, but I was an unscrupulous person. I always felt threatened and always assumed that anyone who was not part of my family or friends had the potential intention to harm me. I was always vigilant and thought three steps ahead, always trying to take into account all eventualities. I wouldn't describe myself as paranoid because many life events shaped me into this person and my brain was just trying to protect me in its way, but I was in a permanent state of stress as a result. I knew that it would still be a lot of work to deal with myself, but I was ready to do so in the coming months.

But now things were looking up, I made a huge leap forward,

and the COVID-19 infection gave me, in retrospect, a huge push forward. I went back to restaurants with my girlfriend and spent more time with my family, I had developed much greater capacities for social life and my best friend booked a forest cabin in the Palatinate and said that we were going on vacation.

I was excited. On the one hand, doubts spread, on the other hand, anticipation. I tried to push all doubts aside and kept visualizing the vacation and how well I would be doing there, I did every day until our departure. I also knew from Richard, who had recently flown to Italy for work, that he had tolerated the trip well, and I classified the Palatinate as less stressful than a flight to Italy, which was also associated with work.

The anticipation outweighed my doubts and on the first of May 2023, it started. A four-hour car ride preceded our vacation, which I mastered better than expected as a passenger, we talked and laughed a lot. I briefly remembered the trip to Hanover, where I had been lying on the back seat with sunglasses and earmuffs, but quickly pushed the thought out of my consciousness. The past had happened, the future unknown and only the here and now mattered. I was doing incredibly well in the Palatinate and, as in Hanover, I noticed that a change of location had a positive influence on my condition. For the first time, I felt a real joy in life again and even though I was very reduced in what I could do physically, we made the best of the time and I found the nature around us indescribably healing. It felt as if a calm had returned to my nervous system.

The only excesses of my illness showed up in my restless sleep, as I woke up several times a night and also increasingly bizarre dreams appeared. One of these dreams from my vacation stayed in my memory. I dreamed that I was out and about in the city with my girlfriend and we were standing in front of a big Ferris wheel. I said to her, "I'm not healthy yet, I can walk around the city with you here, but soon we'll be able to go on the Ferris wheel."

I think this dream made it clear that my subconscious now also believed that I would get well. We used the rest of the holiday to explore our surroundings a bit, and when my best friend went hiking, I stayed in the hut and used the time for my meditation. In the end, there was even a trip to a nearby castle ruin, on the incline that led to it, I felt like I had almost three heart attacks, but with enough breaks, I made it and was overwhelmed by the view that was offered to us.

Throughout the castle ruins, small lizards scurried around and hid in the cracks, where they could be easily observed. They looked like little monitor lizards, and I only noticed afterwards that I was so distracted that I no longer noticed my symptoms.

Back home, I experienced a violent crash after the vacation, which lasted for five days and threw me off track. I recognized the parallels to Hanover and accepted that I would not be able to maintain the level in the long term as in the Palatinate, but would take a step back again. This acceptance made me react much more calmly and made everything more bearable, as I understood more and more for myself how the disease worked.

I was already planning my next vacation for July, which I would spend together with my girlfriend in the Extertal on the border with Lower Saxony. My recovery progressed at a faster pace from that point on than before, and outside of my crash phases, I experienced a gratitude for my life that I had never known before.

I would say that at that time I had 35 per cent of my health, I find it hard to express health subjectively in numbers, but it offers something tangible. Slowly, some strength returned to my body, and whenever I made it, I accompanied my girlfriend shopping, since I often felt bad and I could contribute little to our household (she had recently moved in with me completely), this was a great way not to feel so useless.

When the day came when I carried water from the car to the apartment for the first time, I felt like Mr Universe, it was incredibly exhausting for me, but the point where I was able to let go of the fear of physical activity for the first time. I decided that I was ready to train again, even if the term training sounds a bit bigger than you might think. I started doing movements again with empty barbells, I wanted to get my brain to no longer see sport as a danger, but as something we would do with positivity.

I wouldn't have to be able to push a hundred kilos anymore or have the thickest upper arm and that took a lot of pressure off me. I felt comfortable the way I was and made myself aware that the image other people have of me does not depend on how muscular I am an incredibly liberating feeling. In general, I felt that I wanted my health back, but not my life, I didn't know exactly what my new life, which I wanted to lead at some point, would look like, but I knew that I would have to make a lot of changes.

One night, when I was living through another disturbing dream about my past, there was a kind of aha moment. All of a sudden, I seemed to understand that the dreams that had plagued me for so long might contain the concrete things I would have to face. My brain presented me on a silver platter with the inner conflicts that burdened me. That day, my approach to my dreams changed. I now actively dealt with them and that was anything but easy.

I realized how many fears I had been carrying around with me suppressed for so long and how many toxic relationships I was in. I relived traumatic events in my dreams and during the day I allowed the feelings associated with them and gave them a space, but tried not to let them dominate me. I found dreams that dealt with my moves to be particularly negative, in these I was always a fugitive who tried to run away, but never arrived and was safe.

In this phase, I used many of my capacities to resolve these conflicts and noticeably noticed that more and more burdens fell off my soul. I even have the feeling today that some dreams processed certain key events because after them I made health progress and felt like a big change had occurred.

Richard experienced this the same way as I did and together we stood by each other's side with words and deeds, because often it is enough to say things to be able to let go of them afterwards. In addition, he provided me with new information as he was reading a book on healing trauma and post-traumatic stress disorder, many of the techniques also proved to be extremely useful for me with Long Covid.

Summer had come and with it our holiday near the Lippe Uplands, where I broke new records again, I managed to walk seven thousand steps in one day and climb the Hermann Monument, from which a beautiful view over the forest was possible. I looked into the distance, fourteen months ago I was so ill that I couldn't leave my apartment, now I was standing up here looking out over the valley. I knew that my way would still be long, but I had come a long way.

After we arrived back at the holiday home, I made myself a coffee and sat with my girlfriend on our terrace at the edge of the forest, and although I expected severe symptoms after the day's exertion, nothing happened quite the opposite. While I was stirring my coffee, I said to my friend, "I feel 100 per cent healthy right now."

It was the first moment when I felt completely healthy, my mind was clear and my body was light as a feather, even though this great moment passed, I still caught a glimpse of how great it will be when I am well again. In the evening we drove around by car until late at night and explored nature, it was a perfect holiday and I was almost sad that we had to leave the next day. As usual, a violent temporary crash at home followed, but I found it a little less agonizing than expected, in general, it was noticeable that my adaptation phases became milder. They still hit the first day, but most of the time I felt a little better the following day, I was no longer forced to lie in bed and avoid stimuli until the symptoms subsided, but was able to do small activities mindfully.

However, I had to be particularly careful here, because I still had to take good care of myself and too much activity could easily prolong my crash for a few days. After I recovered, I settled at a level where I was packing an average of 5000 steps a day and my maximum power was around 7000 steps. I was extremely satisfied that there was finally a progression on a physical level. Monitoring my steps could make me feel positive whenever I set a new record, but it could also depress me if I only managed 1000 steps on a bad day, so I decided to let go and deleted the app from my phone. When I was healthy, I never counted my steps either, so I didn't see any benefit in it anymore, I didn't need the visual confirmation of my progress anymore.

As more and more health returned to my life, it was inevitably followed by normal problems. When I was still completely in my cocoon of healing, I did not expose myself to this stress or was not confronted with it at all. But now the time had come when I would take on more responsibility again, and I can tell you, stress was my final boss. Making a phone call, paying a bill or attending an appointment are normal activities that everyone does every day, but for me, they were challenges, a stressful phone call in which I got upset could quickly lead to a flare-up of symptoms. Likewise, unforeseeable events, that life at home can be planned, but life outside in the real world the healthy is not. Richard once said a sentence to me that has remained in my memory to this day:

"Every person can live in two worlds. In the world of the sick, but also the world of the healthy, he can only have one citizenship."

I only understood the importance of this quote at a later point in time. At the moment, I felt like someone with a visa in the world of the healthy, no longer seriously ill, but not healthy either. I spent a lot of time meditating on them after implementing new activities and imagining a sense of security, which helped me incredibly on my way to integrating somewhere on the edge of life. My upward trend was only interrupted when I discovered a wandering flush on my thigh. I must have been bitten by a tick on my last vacation and had this clarified by a dermatologist.

Less than a week later, I received the dreaded message by phone: Lyme disease. Three weeks of antibiotics lay ahead of me and old thought patterns began to come up in me, antibiotics and Long Covid or CFS should not get along at all, that's what I often heard in the groups at that time. Since I didn't feel like sitting there with crippled joints for a few years, there wasn't much to negotiate. Antibiotics were a must. I felt miserable as hell for the next three weeks, I took my medication in the morning and evening and tried to get through the day somehow without falling into too much worry about deterioration.

I succeeded sometimes more, sometimes less well because I was set back in my performance for weeks, but I consoled myself with the thought that even healthy people would not simply put up with several weeks of antibiotics. I started thinking much healthier and didn't want to associate everything with Long Covid anymore. How could I ever get well if I didn't think like a healthy person and made the decision that from now on I would call myself healthy with restrictions? Visually, you could no longer see my illness. I was no longer the pale man with the red eyes I had met in the mirror for so long, but someone who was fighting for his life back. I now proceeded more flexibly and adapted individually to situations. For example, if I had slept badly one night, I would no longer think in the morning that it was due to Long Covid and that now my whole day would be bad. I interrupted the worries and said to myself: Everyone sleeps badly sometimes, that's part of a healthy life.

When I got dizzy, I interrupted my thoughts about this and said to myself: Oh, I must have drunk too little water today. Even if that wasn't true, it was all about tricking my brain and I managed to do that better and better over time. My entire world of thoughts slowly detached itself from the patterns that brought everything into connection with the disease to try, that brain is always looking for danger and if you let it, it will always find something and then see itself confirmed in the fact that we are in danger.

Due to my increasingly strong emotional stability, my physical resilience grew rapidly, things that threw me off track a year ago I now did almost casually. Just drive to Edeka and do a big shopping? No problem, there was even time for a relaxed conversation with the cashier. During the activity, the symptoms often faded into the background and only flared up afterwards, but conscious breaks had a soothing effect on me again, not like at the beginning of the disease, where you sleep and are almost more exhausted after waking up than the day before. I usually lay down to meditate throughout the day, sometimes for ten minutes, sometimes for half an hour, depending on how long it took me to calm down. I deliberately said to myself: I just changed tyres, it was exhausting and it's okay that I need a break now. Every healthy person needs breaks.

I tried to keep the balance between activity and breaks, which sometimes proved difficult as I felt an incredibly strong drive to want to do it all. I often had to consciously slow myself down not to go beyond my limits too often, even if I treated myself mentally like a healthy person, I still had to be mindful and respect my physical limits. The whole thing is like dancing on a tightrope, and I've lost my balance and crashed at least a hundred times, but I never gave up and each crash made me come back stronger.

The whole principle was extremely simple. Too much stress

was followed by symptoms, which I met with serenity and took it easy for some time and after a few days, my limits shifted upwards. It was always the same cycle from the beginning. My nervous system always needed its time to adapt to new things, and most of the time I dreamed of the activity I had previously carried out that same night, as if my brain were consciously asking me if we were safe.

In autumn, many of the symptoms slowly lost their intensity, the muscle twitches that could appear randomly in any part of my body disappeared, and even my feet and hands, which were always cold, returned to normal temperature. My food sensitivity disappeared completely and the feeling of alienation did not appear at all from that point on. In November 2023, I went on vacation again with my girlfriend, again to the same place in the Extertal. Since a few months had passed since our last stay and we were in the same place, I was able to measure my progression well and it was enormous.

We went on excursions, and explorations and even took part in a castle tour in Lower Saxony. During my first vacation we also spent wonderful days here, but this time we were much more active, I was not afraid of physical activity or the resulting symptoms, I let myself be carried away completely by the joy and noticed that if I distracted myself strongly from an activity, i.e. did not do it consciously, this triggered fewer reactions than if I focused on it.

Walking in pairs was much better than alone because then my head began to create worrying thoughts, but in pairs, I was distracted by the conversation and did not even notice the distance I had covered. I experienced a change in my symptoms, while at the beginning of the disease, the focus was more on the physical in the form of weakness, pain and circulatory disorders, the symptomatology now changed more to an emotional level. When I went beyond my limits, there were no more severe physical reactions that tied me to the bed and tormented me, I felt more burnt out and joyless on those days, but this was much better to bear than lying in bed with a pulse of 120 and just staring at the wall because everything else would overstimulate you.

At the beginning of my illness, physical exertion was not possible and harmful, but now that changed and I had to do more and more to push my physical limits higher. I spent many hours of meditation breaking old thought patterns: I spoke to myself and explained to myself that effort was once harmful to me, but now I was allowed to let go of the part of me that was conditioned to always warn me.

Recovery is a process that does not work linearly and every new physical challenge is followed by a mental one, and since the body always follows the mind, the mind must heal and the body will do the same. My immune system also seemed to normalize more and more at the same time, as slowly but surely the flu-like symptoms were much less common, and I no longer suffered from sinus or sore throat as often as before.

Increasing my physical performance had now become my priority, I built in time to go for a walk two to three times a week, and I consciously chose well-known places that I associated with positive memories.

Over time, I improved more and more. The first time I walked 10,000 steps, a violent boomerang of exhaustion and brain fog followed, but within a week I recovered and repeated my record. I was obsessed with reaching the 12,000 steps, but I was much more careful than I used to be. I came to accept that I was not achieving goals or not as quickly as I wanted to, and with this acceptance, my quality of life continued to increase. I exerted myself when I could and withdrew when my body demanded rest and recovery and as my feeling for it got better and better, the symptoms became milder and milder. Vacation was an insane lever for me that I could use to make progress, if the whole thing had been a game, I would say that I reached a new level after each vacation, which was reflected in improvements within a very short time. With the same friend whom I had already accompanied to the Palatinate Forest, the next holiday in nature was on the agenda, we drove to Schleusingen in the Thuringian Forest.

I always experienced nature as very healing and everything in me came to rest, the inner child in me was thrilled by the almost endless forests and castles that were enthroned on the peaks. A castle ruin with the name Osterburg was our first destination, it was now time to overcome an incline. The ascent was short but intense, since we did not use the official path but a beaten path, we soon found ourselves in a very steep environment and here the fearful thoughts struck.

Can I do it?

Am I overdoing it right now and getting a relapse?

I gathered my courage and climbed the clearing where the castle was located, while my friend was still exploring the forest, I had to take a break, I sat down at the old well of the castle, which was sealed with a grate and while panting trying to recover, I was suddenly distracted by its depth. I picked up a stone and let it fall into the darkness, about fifteen meters I mumbled when I suddenly realized that I had recovered. I was amazed and pleased about my quick regeneration and visited another castle on the same day, which was also located in an elevated position.

In the evening I accompanied my friend on his hike until I noticed that now was the time for me to turn around and rest. I slept extremely restlessly the night and the next day I felt like I was slain, not like the first days of my illness but still so that it worried me. After breakfast, I realized that my friend was also exhausted and had to nibble on the effort of the previous day. At that moment I knew that I was allowed to let go. The exhaustion was not the product of my illness, but a result of our effort.

My friend, who is blessed with the best of health, was also exhausted. I thought a lot about the fact that exhaustion is something normal that everyone knows in their life and not every day that you feel weak and powerless means that the disease has returned. I had to dissolve this thought pattern, but I knew that the process would take some time, just like everything else. Patience is an essential virtue. 2023 was now slowly coming to an end and even though it was a difficult year for me, I looked back on many wonderful experiences.

Chapter 6
New life

What does a new life mean? I think if you asked a hundred people this question, you would get a hundred different answers, so I tried to figure out for myself what my new life should be. I thought about what made me sick and didn't want me in my life anymore: stress, unresolved conflicts, self-hatred and doubt, toxic relationships and professional activities that didn't fulfil me.

At that time, I often imagined my future self sitting next to me and telling me what a fulfilled life I would lead in the future. Many of my goals were long-term, but there were also those that I could tackle in the short term. It was time to settle down, and I actively started looking for a new home where my girlfriend and I would live. I discovered a condominium in need of renovation and decided to buy it, since my girlfriend's father owned a construction company, the renovation was not a challenge for us.

But I took every chance to help the craftsmen, it was the first time that I did physical work again, from hauling material to laying the floor. I helped where I could and found that I could now almost keep up with healthy people for a while.

During this time, I talked a lot with my girlfriend's father, who asked me if I would help with something in the office from January 2024. I was still a bit anxious about working since I didn't have any strong economic pressure, I wanted to take at least another year for my full recovery, but I said yes anyway. I knew at that time that I didn't want to go back to my job at school, in general, I didn't want to work as an employee anymore. I wanted to become self-employed, it sounds paradoxical, but I knew that I would have more stress as a boss, but I could also regulate it better. If I meditate in my office, no one could reprimand me for it. I knew how to negotiate and approached my friend's father and rejected his offer afterwards.

On further inquiries, I denied everything for the first time, until the time came when he approached me and asked if I wanted to set up a GmbH with him. I had achieved my goal. I now had a new home and a perspective and my strategy of recovery changed from that point on. I now had to pick up the pace and do more and more. I did not neglect my meditations, but it was time to give up my citizenship in the world of the sick and to switch body and mind to the world of the healthy.

My weeks filled up more and more with appointments, conversations here, negotiations there, plans about founding the company and another five-hour meeting the next day. Two years ago I was very ill and my brain frog made simple conversations impossible, now I sat for hours in meetings with managing directors and people from the construction industry. These meetings triggered severe symptoms at the beginning, but I was happy because to trigger these violent phases, a meeting lasting several hours was now necessary. My level was now almost at that of a person who had never suffered from Long Covid, I knew that from now on it would only take time until I had fully regenerated.

Since my return to work tied up a lot of my capacities, I had to give up many things that I liked to do before, but sometimes it makes more sense to leave things out and then make progressions in other areas. I stopped my walks to have more energy for my appointments because at that time I was so exhausted in the evening that I was usually in bed from 7:30 p.m. onwards. But it was no longer the pathological fatigue that I was experiencing, but real fatigue from the day. I was absolutely happy and usually fell asleep around 10 p.m. and then slept through my seven to eight hours, the symptom that tormented me the most was gone, I no longer had trouble sleeping through the night, and I didn't need melatonin anymore.

My dreams changed and I experienced positive and hopeful dreams of a healthy future, everything in my body, but also my environment, slowly normalized and the disease went more and more into the background.

Richard, who was always on the same level as me, gave me a

tip that would further speed up my recovery. My healing was not linear, but in retrospect, I made more and more reliable progress from month to month. I usually proceeded very analytically and planned my steps carefully. Richard suggested to me that it was now time to give up this security a bit, of course, he did not advise me to push my body to the extreme, but simply to slowly dismantle the caution I had acquired.

I knew he was right, but when you were sick for two years and always had to be careful not to go too far beyond your limits, you were conditioned to it. I was also in contact with someone who had CFS a few years ago and has fully recovered, and he also told me that his journey could be easily divided into three phases: the phase of rest, the phase of mindful increase and the push phase back to life.

I would now be in this phase and would have to step on the gas pedal to do the rest. I now decided to tackle my health construction sites, which had accumulated independently of my illness. My teeth needed treatment and even though the visit to the dentist was not pleasant, I no longer wanted to run away from taking responsibility for my health. I made an appointment by phone and explained to my dentist why I had to postpone the treatment for two years. She reacted sympathetically to my situation and treated my molar tooth, which had lost its filling.

To my regret, it was discovered that I rubbed away a few millimetres of my teeth as part of my illness and my temporomandibular joint was affected. A root inflamed tooth also had to be extracted and elsewhere I needed an implant and a splint in case the grinding should come back.

I knew that I would spend many hours in the dentist's chair for the next few months, and I was a bit afraid of the injection, as I had often read in the past that it worked with adrenaline, which could be very unpleasant with the disease. My worries turned out to be unfounded, in one week an inflammation forced me to go to the dentist three times and with each local anaesthesia nothing happened, except that my pulse shot up a bit beforehand.

Even the extraction of my molar tooth with the following antibiotic did not cause any further problems. I had overcome my fear, which came from the beginning of the disease, so the next thing I did was to see an ophthalmologist and get new glasses.

I was very happy to be able to go to doctors who could help me. I think hardly anyone likes to go to the doctor, but when you were so sick that you couldn't make it to the practice, it was now a great feeling to keep these appointments.

I started exercising almost every day and enjoyed my life. I developed an acceptance that my healing would take as long as it takes.

My quality of life had returned and living at 85 percent was quite fulfilling. I started my sport by training my calves every day and over the weeks I began to integrate other muscle groups. I increased slowly but steadily and built in more and more exercises until I was able to do a full-fledged workout again. Most of the time, I listened to calming music while exercising or meditating and paid a lot of attention to my breathing. I was amazed at the speed at which I was building up strength and endurance again. Muscle memory was my ally, and as long as I managed to keep my nervous system calm, I was able to train hard.

However, I completely let go of the pressure that I had to be the strongest or the broadest, the sport should now enrich my life and promote my health and not trigger more stress in me as before. In general, I would describe the sport as a kind of turbo that drove my recovery. In the past, physical exertion would have been harmful, but now it was exactly what I needed to get back to the next level. In principle, I was able to do everything I wanted again. I went on many trips with my girlfriend and tried new things, and I also started to write down my story. This was not always easy for me, as the first chapters in particular were associated with the fact that I consciously put myself back in this time, but the thought of encouraging other people always pleased me while writing.

I enjoyed social activities more than before. I used to be always stressed, but now I sat for hours with my friends or went to a restaurant with my girlfriend. The feeling of being rushed, which I often felt in the past with such things, had disappeared, it was replaced by joie de vivre and happiness. Time passed and I invested a lot of time in planning and founding the company, I believed that the serenity I now possessed was a skill that would be of particular benefit to me in the future as a managing director. Stress had become a part of my life again, but it didn't accumulate as much as it used to, as I now had plenty of techniques to relax.

I have also learned to admit a lot to myself and to represent my opinion, to my initial surprise, most people react rather positively when you explain to them objectively why you don't want things or why you have a different opinion. The power of saying no has been essential for me on my road to recovery. I had to do this many hundreds of times, often even though I would have liked to do this or that, but I knew it wouldn't have been good for me. I also lost the fear of rejection. We are all human beings and everyone wants to be loved, perhaps also because evolutionarily the expulsion from a group used to result in certain death.

But I got rid of the illusion that what other people would think of me mattered. I lived in such a way that I could look in the mirror and be satisfied with myself, and I think that's actually what counts in life, not wanting to impress strangers who you don't like or want to participate in their stupid habitus. I decided to go to the sea with my girlfriend to spend some nice days with her. We set off and started our journey, after which a lot of work would await both of us, but I learned that a lot of work and stress must always be accompanied by relaxation and balance. We rode our bikes for 30 kilometres and crossed a large dune that built up in front of us, when we had climbed the height, the white beach spread out in front of us and about 200 meters away the sea began.

I took off my shoes and went to the water. The cold seawater enclosed my feet while my gaze wandered into the endless distance. I had arrived at my destination and at the same time, it was the beginning of a new journey. I was reborn and as endless as the ocean that lay before me were the possibilities of my new life.

We were about to start our company and plan our future together, we talked a lot about getting married, about what it would be like to buy a house and have children. I felt deep gratitude that the disease came into my life and shaped me into the person I am now; from the depths of my being, a sentence forced its way into my consciousness: "I will never see the sea again."

END

Thanks

If you were to ask me today what has helped me the most on my twenty-five-month journey to recovery, I would answer, "Acceptance." The acceptance of having lost one's health and no longer being able to take care of oneself is not easy to accept and yet necessary, as denial of the situation is often accompanied by a further deterioration of the situation. When we understand that acceptance is not synonymous with a task, we understand that we must first admit to ourselves where we stand before things can get better.

Many people I met did not manage to get well and lost themselves in a vortex of physical symptoms and fear that took them further and further.

These people have my sympathy from the bottom of my heart because I know how quickly you can lose control and succumb to the overpowering disease. I lost a lot of contact with people I liked and who, in my eyes, didn't deserve to die of the disease. I am grateful that I have found my way back to life, but I do not have the power to heal other people. The path that was right for me can be the wrong one for other people. My truth about the disease does not have to be the truth of another sufferer, but even if it was only my faith – I have become healthy.

In conclusion, I would like to say that there are many people to whom I feel gratitude, as they helped me on my way and were always there for me when I needed them, but I also feel a profound gratitude towards illness. It came into my life and at first glance took away everything important, but it was also the illness who made me grow, because without it I would not be where I am today. I live my life more consciously and happily than I ever did before. It's the little things in life that I can now enjoy. I learned an inner balance, and the confidence in myself now seems almost inexhaustible.

I was never an esotericist or in any other way spiritual or religious, but what I went through made me a better person. The path was incredibly hard and I experienced countless setbacks, disappointments and fears, often I wanted to give up, but finally went the way to the end.

I thank all the people I had the pleasure of meeting and who accompanied me on my way, my family and my girlfriend, Rufus, Deniz, Matyas, Béla and Rafael. And I wish every reader of my book only the best and health from the bottom of my heart.

Christoph D. Theissen

www.ingramcontent.com/pod-product-compliance
Lightning Source LLC
Chambersburg PA
CBHW071958210526
45479CB00003B/985